The Physician's Survival Guide for the Hospital

The Physician's Survival Guide for the Hospital

Let the Hospital Work for You

SAMUEL H. STEINBERG, PH.D.

iUniverse, Inc.
New York   Bloomington

The Physician's Survival Guide for the Hospital
Let the Hospital Work for You

Copyright © 2006, 2008 by Samuel H. Steinberg

All rights reserved. No part of this book may be used or reproduced by any means, graphic, electronic, or mechanical, including photocopying, recording, taping or by any information storage retrieval system without the written permission of the publisher except in the case of brief quotations embodied in critical articles and reviews.

iUniverse Star
an iUniverse, Inc. imprint

iUniverse books may be ordered through booksellers or by contacting:

iUniverse
1663 Liberty Drive
Bloomington, IN 47403
www.iuniverse.com
1-800-Authors (1-800-288-4677)

Because of the dynamic nature of the Internet, any Web addresses or links contained in this book may have changed since publication and may no longer be valid. The views expressed in this work are solely those of the author and do not necessarily reflect the views of the publisher, and the publisher hereby disclaims any responsibility for them.

ISBN: 978-1-60528-026-4 (pbk)
ISBN: 978-0-595-63157-5 (ebk)

Printed in the United States of America

To my family.
Your encouragement and support mean everything.

Contents

Foreword... ix
Introduction.. xi

Part I — Everyday Business

Chapter 1 Activities of Daily Living: How to Take Charge of Orienting Yourself to the Hospital................3

Chapter 2 Learning the Rules and Complying with the Important Ones.................................8

Chapter 3 Who Is in Charge? Adopt an Administrator........10

Chapter 4 What Committees Should I Serve On and Why?.....................................12

Chapter 5 Working with Residents, Hospitalists, and Intensivists..................................15

Part II — Necessary Financial Knowledge

Chapter 6 How Does the Hospital Make Money?............21

Chapter 7 Understanding the Operating Budget.............25

Chapter 8 Capital Equipment: Getting What You Need......29

Part III — Understanding the Institutional Environment

Chapter 9 What Is a Health System, and Should I Care?......35

Chapter 10 What Does a Trustee Do?.......................40

CHAPTER 11   What Does Nonprofit Status Really Mean? 44

Part IV   Topics of General Interest

CHAPTER 12   Academic Practice versus Private Practice.......... 49

CHAPTER 13   What Do I Need to Know about Information Technology?............................... 53

CHAPTER 14   Hospital-Physician Integration: Making a Deal 58

CHAPTER 15   Oh, No! Not Another Quality Improvement Program..................................... 62

CHAPTER 16   A Practical and Strategic Evaluation of Your Practice 66

Part V   Closing Thoughts

Appendix... 75

Foreword

Practicing medicine is not getting any easier. Neither is running a hospital. Bringing the two efforts together successfully becomes more complex with each new medical advance, governmental regulation, and shift in the marketplace. Being effective in this environment requires the skills of a scientist, a psychologist, and a politician.

The practice of medicine in a hospital is not something easily learned in a classroom. One learns through trial and error. Seasoned physicians and administrators have learned some of their most important lessons from their failures.

Success in health-care delivery today requires an ability to balance quality, service, and efficiency. Outcomes are increasingly transparent, and managed-care organizations, employers, and consumers are more demanding. Timelines for producing results have been shortened. With these increasing demands, the contemporary physician needs all the advice and formulas for achieving results that can be found.

In this book, Steinberg shares more than thirty years of experience and wisdom that bring clarity to physician-hospital relations. His observations and lessons are invaluable for physicians wishing to improve the efficiency and effectiveness of their time spent in the hospital. Most importantly, he demystifies the activities that go on behind administrative walls and lets physicians in on the secrets that will make them successful.

Steinberg's writing is focused on working with people, particularly physicians, which is something he has always been noted for. The ability to understand the perspectives of both the physician and the administrator is the key to being successful in our business, and he has that ability. This book should serve as a useful companion for all who want to challenge their own thinking and learn from a master. As you read this, I hope you expand your perspective and learn to increase the value of the time you spend in the hospital.

David J. Shulkin, MD
President and Chief Executive Officer,
Beth Israel Health System
New York, New York

Introduction

The Problem

You would think that physicians and hospitals go together like peanut butter and jelly. Doctors need hospitals, and hospitals need doctors. Common sense, right? Unfortunately, it has become obvious to me in thirty-plus years of health-care administration that this is not the case. Many physicians have a difficult time functioning in the hospital environment, and administrators are continually frustrated by physician decision making and behavior. The underlying cause of this is poor quality communication between physicians and administrators that sometimes borders on mistrust and skepticism.

Many times, I have observed discussions on how this situation can be improved, and the recommendation I hear most often is to hold for residents a lecture or a day of events devoted to how to succeed in hospital practice. In fact, the Accreditation Commission for Graduate Medical Education has recently included business knowledge concepts as one of the six general competencies that residents must master. Although this may benefit residents, and whether it does is questionable, it does nothing to focus on hospital practice. Training sessions are held with little or no impact, and everyone feels better about attempting to do something. Most physicians can benefit from a discussion of the business realities of health care, but this does not begin to touch on the issue of improving how physicians practice in the hospital.

I suspect that anyone from outside the health-care system reading this must wonder, "What is Sam talking about?" How can it be that physicians and hospital administrators do not communicate well when they work together every day? Yet, those of us who experience the situation on a daily basis can tell you that although these two groups may work together, they exist in their own self-imposed separate worlds. This is not an issue reserved for the health-care field, since members of many other segments of our society—officers and enlisted people in the military services, for example—also experience this subdivision. Doctors socialize with one another, nurses, and other clinicians in their gatherings, but these gatherings rarely include administrators. Administrators operate in a similar fashion. Starting from their higher education, administrators and health-care professionals' lives are very separate. Throughout medical or graduate school, there can be little interaction. It is not a surprise that both parties are often frustrated, and overcoming these frustrations would be the best way to improve everyone's performance and satisfaction.

Health-care administrators are frustrated by the seeming inability or unwillingness of physicians to practice as the administrators desire in the hospital environment, and physicians are equally frustrated with what often seem to be silly rules; with the difficulty in getting things done for their patients; and with the never-ending calls, e-mails, and correspondence they must endure from the administrators regarding the things they are not doing or are doing incorrectly. Given that these are all smart people and that they all are focused on patient care, it remains difficult to comprehend why these conflicts and frustrations continue to occur in nearly every hospital throughout the United States.

As I have been writing this book, and discussing the issues with both physicians and administrative colleagues, it has become apparent to me that the quality of the professional relationships among these parties is at fault. Mistrust, poor communication, and the ever-changing nature of the health-care delivery system contribute to a focus on their own needs by the members of each profession, rather than a focus on the mission of the organization and on the needs of patients. Having to meet one's regulatory and bureaucratic requirements while dealing with the new consumerist patient and fighting over a shrinking income does not promote collegiality or improve the quality of the work being performed.

The Solution: Sharing the Secrets

My contribution to solving this problem is the creation of this manual for hospital physicians and administrators. As an experienced hospital administrator with more than three decades of experience working with physicians, I can provide simple, direct, and clear answers to the many questions physicians have and can write with a high degree of knowledge regarding the day-to-day operations of a hospital.

I intend this manual to enable physicians to do what they need for their patients and to help them manage their day while devoting as little time as possible to time-wasting, non-patient-care activities. This manual applies to both young physicians and seasoned practitioners. In this manual I help administrators to find how best to work with their clinician colleagues, how to smooth the frustrations of their daily interactions, and how to avoid much of the non-value-added time and energy they currently spend on recurring problems related to physician practice.

How is this possible? Understanding the rules of successful coexistence between physicians and administrators, I focus sharply in this manual on the knowledge and skills physicians must learn to function in the hospital, and I give straightforward guidelines for accomplishing essential tasks and for ignoring those things that are not really necessary. For example, though all hospitals are responsible for orienting new medical staff members to their facility and for delineating the staff members' responsibilities, few hospitals actually do this well. Administrators do not seem to understand what physicians really need to know and why many physicians find these orientations useless, feeling that they are left to their own devices to learn informally from their colleagues. For example, physicians need to know practical information, such as how to write orders and how and where to chart. They must be able to complete their billing requirements and medical records, and they need to understand what the hospital's rules and regulations are regarding paging and emergency situations. More often than not, physicians learn this information through trial and error and become angry and disappointed in their hospital practice early on. Hospital administrators become upset with newly appointed physicians as well, not realizing that they, the administrators, could have eliminated these trial-and-error problems with proper education for the new physicians. Unfortunately, this situation gives rise to the suspicions and mistrust that often spring up between physicians and hospital administrators.

My goal here is to provide physicians with the knowledge they need to have about how to orient themselves and function on a daily basis and regarding what is going on around them, who is running the show, and where best to spend their most limited resource—their time. Equally important is for hospital administrators to understand what physicians look at, how they perceive matters, and what issues are of concern to them. Physicians need to know what committees are worth serving on, what the Board of Trustees does and how the board's decisions affect patients, what is really important on those endless financial statements, and how can they position themselves for success and optimal patient care. Ultimately, physicians need to understand what their practice is worth to the hospital, both financially and strategically, so that they can focus and leverage their activities to their best advantage. These understandings and others can be developed through straight talk and the inside information that physicians must know in order to be confident that they are utilizing their hospital time wisely.

Each chapter highlights what physicians really need to know and what they must actually do in order to be victorious in the daily battles with administrators, various bureaucrats, and all those regulators who are trying to control physicians' behavior or even take away their ability to care for patients. There are no more secrets: the real stuff that you need to know is provided here. Armed with the proper knowledge, both physicians and administrators will be able to fulfill their mission, manage their schedules, and minimize their wasted time.

In reviewing my philosophical approach to the topics discussed here, I have found that this book has become a personal journey. One cannot provide opinions regarding the best way to perform a task without reflecting on the experiences that shaped the values and beliefs behind the opinions. The health-care delivery system has changed dramatically over the past thirty-five years, not all for the better. Although medical knowledge and technology have exploded over that time, the image of the physician has suffered. Patients' rights and consumerism have become societal values, and this has contributed to the erosion of trust in the physician-patient relationship. Throughout this period, health-care practitioners have struggled to evolve and adapt, sometimes not successfully. Physicians are viewed by patients as more interested in monetary rewards and business development than in patient care, nurses choose not to wear uniforms in their quest for professional autonomy, everyone in the hospital setting has multiple sets of initials after his or her name, and patients are often confused about who is taking care of them. It is no wonder that patients seek greater knowledge and self-reliance rather than trust old Dr. Welby to make the best decision for them. Dr. Welby doesn't exist anymore, and we are all confused about who has our best interests at heart. This situation cannot be allowed to persist, and a secondary theme of this book is the need for physicians to clarify their roles as the unbiased leaders of the health-care system and take charge of the system's future. Improving how physicians work in the hospital setting is one step toward achieving this aim.

PART I
Everyday Business

1

Activities of Daily Living: How to Take Charge of Orienting Yourself to the Hospital

I have never met anyone starting a new job who is not a bit nervous about it. Finding out where everything is and determining whom you need to know are among the most uncomfortable aspects of beginning a new job. In fact, I am convinced that many of us choose not to change positions or employers because we are just at ease with where we are. Getting up to speed in a new hospital position can take many months or even a year, so anything that speeds up this process will be beneficial to patient care and to our collective desire to do a good job.

Starting a new position at a hospital is likely to be one of the most frustrating things you will ever have to do in your professional life. But if done well, it can be one of the most useful and beneficial tasks you accomplish as a new physician, and you can ease yourself into your new environment smoothly and make your daily functioning effortless. If you transition into your position poorly, which is much more typical, you will be constantly bombarded with hospital administrators' demands and threats that accuse you of failing to perform adequately.

Orientation

Most hospitals have an orientation program for new physicians. Often, the orientation is stratified by what position you will be taking, with senior physicians getting a lot of attention and junior physicians getting almost none. Your status as a full-time hospital employee or as a volunteer physician will also be a factor here, with full-timers getting significant attention and volunteers (physicians who are not on the payroll) getting little time or attention.

Employed physicians will be given a great deal of information regarding rules and regulations, salary, and benefits and may even be provided some orientation to the physical facility itself. Sometimes this can take an entire day, and attendance is usually mandatory. Frequently, if you actually do get to this program, it is boring and full of jargon, and the orientation leaders pile on a bunch of thick manuals for you to read (as if that will ever happen!). If you make it through the entire program, you sign some affidavit swearing that you now know everything you need to know to function in the hospital (in case something bad happens in the future, they can wave this form at you to show that the mistake you made is your fault), and you are free to forget everything and misplace the manuals as soon as you leave. I have never met any physicians who thought their orientation was an unqualified success and worth the time—hence, my belief that you should orient yourself.

Taking Charge of Orientation

A better process than hospital-organized orientation, in my opinion, revolves around focusing on what you need to know to practice in the hospital and take care of your patients. Start with the medical staff office. The people there verify that you are licensed and have all the documents you need to be credentialed to practice. If your file is missing something, they will help you get that missing documentation. They know whom to contact at the state medical license bureau and every other organization that might impact your ability to practice as quickly as possible. They are your friends, and they will be so amazed that you are reaching out to them that they will bend over backwards to help you. This means that you will be able to begin work quickly and start work without having people all over you on a daily basis asking for a form or a diploma. Insurers will also pay you sooner if you become credentialed quickly.

> **Physician tip:** Carry your paperwork around. There's no better way to meet people and develop relationships.

Admissions

The next stop is the Admissions office, where the staff is in charge of getting your patients into the hospital and assigning them a comfortable room. These people can make you look like a hero to your patients; bad rooms on bad floors are always available, but the good ones are hard to find, and admissions staff know where patients are happy and well cared for and where they are not. If you take the time to meet with the admissions staff, they will immediately identify you as an attending physician who cares and will tell your patients what a good physician you are. It's all about their perception of you.

If you ask the admissions staff, "What do I need to know in order to be successful here?" (you should ask everyone you meet at the hospital this same question), the staff will tell you whom else to meet and will even take you there if you request. Again, because these folks rarely get visits from new physicians, they will always remember you and help you and your patients whenever possible. Make sure to get copies of all available admission forms and patient-information brochures or pamphlets. Remember that these materials were written by the people you are speaking with, and compliment the staff on the look of the materials when you promise to read the information. (In fact, the materials are worth reading since your patients will do so.) When you get that list of everyone that the admissions staff members think you should meet, be certain to write down the name of the admissions director so that you can throw it around. (Name-dropping is a key habit for the successful physician—more on that later.)

> **Physician tip: Treat everyone you meet as a peer. They are professionals too.**

Nursing

Your next visit will be to the office of the Director of Nursing. This person is very important to see, but he or she is often in meetings all day, so make an appointment if necessary. Being proactive in meeting the nursing leadership will resonate throughout the entire nursing department, and no department in the hospital has a better grapevine than nursing. After physicians, nurses are the people most often asked for their opinions of a doctor, so it is incumbent upon you to interact well with your nursing colleagues. When you meet with the director, ask lots of questions about staffing ratios, the nursing organization structure (both on the units and at the administrative level), and request a tour of all the facilities you will need to know about for your particular practice and specialty. Nothing enhances the nursing director's status like taking a physician around, and nothing improves the physician's reputation in the hospital like being seen as a friend and supporter of nursing. (Keep in mind that the opposite is also true, and the nursing department can sink your reputation faster than any other group can.) Even if your physician colleagues don't like you, when the nurses speak well of you, your reputation is safe, particularly with the administration, which listens closely to nursing.

> **Administrator tip:** Make all these offices visible and easy to find. Stop hiding them in the basement.

Medical Records

The last of the absolutely required visits of your self-orientation program is to Medical Records. Like the staff in the other offices already discussed, these folks can make or break your reputation as well as increase your misery level. You must understand that the money trail begins with the medical records and that the surest way to get in trouble is to be late in completing your medical records or to fail to complete them in the required fashion. A bill for an inpatient stay cannot go out until the medical record is completed, and a bill for an outpatient service cannot be sent until you complete your part of the record. Make completing your charts or operative notes a daily activity, in the hospital as well as in your own office. The finances of the entire institution, as well as the hospital's accreditation and licensure status, have more to do with accurate, timely, and complete medical record documentation than with anything else. Even your own malpractice profile can be impacted as much by your handling of the medical records as by your interaction with your patients. Remember: if it does not appear on the record, it did not happen. Further, if something appears on the record late, it makes the medical record staff crazy, and they will make you crazy in turn, contacting you every day and even potentially suspending your hospital privileges. The quickest way to become perceived as a problem physician is to be a medical record delinquent!

Also, find out from the medical record staff how to meet the federal and state compliance standards in place at your hospital; this information is often available in template fashion specifically drawn up for your specialty or department. Find out what you need to include on the chart to determine the level of service for billing purposes, and chart on your inpatients every day they are in the hospital. There may be guidelines in existence here; ask about those. Physicians get ranked by such things as insurer-denied days, delinquent records, and lengths of stay beyond what is normal for your type of patients, and these are all the wrong lists to get your name on. Work closely with the medical record staff starting on your first day in order to become known as a physician who is interested in these indicators and who will be a leader in helping administration move the medical staff toward being successful in these problem areas. This is time well spent and will make your professional life more satisfying and less frustrating.

Everything Else

After meeting with what I call the "Big 4" (medical staff office, admissions, nursing, and medical records), list all hospital departments that have a role in caring for your patients. The goal is to visit every area your patients will see, from parking to discharge. Depending on your specialty, this might include the operating rooms and the departments of Anesthesia, Radiology, Pathology, and several others. Schedule some time with each of these departments or functions after putting them in priority order based on your needs. Check them off as you make your visits and try to complete all the visits before you start working at the hospital. This is not always possible, but make the visits as quickly as you can. This well-spent time will establish you as a smart person who cares about everyone who helps you care for your patients. More importantly, whenever your patients tell you about a good service or a problem area, you can tell them that you are familiar with that office or department and that you will look into any problems. Your patients will benefit greatly from your actions, and your daily routine will be easier and more productive.

Administrator tip: Have you visited these places lately?

2

Learning the Rules and Complying with the Important Ones

Hospitals are built upon rules. Many rules are imposed upon the hospital by federal and state authorities, some are the result of standards of practice in your community, and others are reflective of custom and history at particular hospitals. Sorting them out and determining which ones are really necessary to follow can save you a lot of time and effort and also can keep you out of trouble.

This can be a particularly frustrating area for physicians; administrators need to spend more time making these documents more user-friendly and consistently up to date.

Medical Staff Bylaws

Let's start by considering the medical staff bylaws and the rules and regulations. These two documents were likely in that pile of stuff given to you at your orientation or when you first started. You probably only glanced through them, since they can be lengthy and full of perhaps uninteresting information. Many physicians misplace these policies or put them on that shelf for things they will read when they have nothing else to do. If no one gave you these manuals, you can pick them up at the medical staff office.

First look at the rules and regulations, which are usually featured in a separate document at the end of the bylaws. The bylaws themselves are only for reading when you get in trouble and need to know what the procedures are for getting out of said trouble. Since you are reading this book, it is unlikely that this will happen to you, so you can concentrate on the specific things you must know about admitting procedures, your responsibilities to your patient, and the day-to-day activities and duties that you must deal with. If you have properly followed the steps in chapter 1, reading the rules and regulations will reinforce what you learned from those office visits and may even help you make sense of information that was not quite clear. (By the way, if your hospital does not have up-to-date bylaws and rules and regulations, you may want to question why they are out of date, since that may be a sign of a less than competent administration.) The document should offer succinct statements of procedures to follow, should be updated annually, and should not be too lengthy. Read it, keep it handy, and refer to it when needed. Make notes directly on the document as issues arise. It is your friend.

> **Administrator tip:** Update these documents annually. Keep them relevant and useful.

Keeping Up

Beyond the rules and regulations, you will be confronted with a never-ending stream of information that mostly does not apply to you. My advice is to pile it on that shelf I mentioned earlier and, using the same techniques you learned in medical school, remember where the pile is but not what is in it. In the same way that medical knowledge changes so quickly that no human being can keep up, Medicare rules, federal and state regulations, accreditation standards, and the like are also constantly changing, and studying them in detail is not worth a lot of your time. In fact, if the hospital thinks information is important for you to know (i.e., if it could affect their cash flow negatively), they will highlight it for you. Hospitals actually pay people to read this stuff, and you will get many e-mails and memos about specific behaviors or processes that you must adopt or change. As noted later, knowing which e-mails and notices deserve your attention is a skill in itself, a skill worth learning. In any event, concentrate on the things highlighted in this manual, and rest assured you will hear about any legal, regulatory, or accreditation matter that could affect you or get you or the hospital into legal trouble.

> **Administrator tip:** Not everything you send out is important. Highlight those things that are critical.

3

Who Is in Charge? Adopt an Administrator

You must first understand that no one is really in charge of everything that goes on in the hospital. Many physicians who practice there are likely not on the payroll and may practice at several institutions. Administration, the board of trustees, and the medical staff leadership all have a lot to say, but they don't always control the day-to-day activity in the hospital. Nurses and doctors on the floors often have more to say about what really goes on, particularly on the second and third shifts. (One thing hospital execs learn early is to not wander around at night in the hospital; you will see things you don't want to know about.)

The most critical thing to know here, in my view, is that physicians spend significant time interacting only with other physicians and this severely limits their knowledge of the hospital. They go to meetings with doctors, socialize mostly with doctors, and even live near other doctors, sometimes forming very upscale doctor neighborhoods in well-to-do sections of cities and towns. I suspect that social scientists would say that this is normal and natural behavior driven by instinct, but it results in a limited range of information and can cause dysfunction in the hospital setting.

Although this self-segregation is often comforting and easy to develop, it leaves the new physician at the mercy of other physicians' biases and those physicians' own limited knowledge of what is going on and who is in control of their hospital. The best way to overcome this limited vision is to enlarge the circle of people you interact with, particularly to include hospital administrative folk and even trustees (more on who they are in another chapter). Some physicians include nurses and other clinical and technical people in their daily interactions, but have little or no contact with the administrators in their department or institution.

> **Physician tip: Stop those boring "doctors only" parties. Be the catalyst in broadening your colleagues' focus.**

I recommend strongly that a new physician meet with as many administrators as possible. Go to the hospital administrative offices (often quite well hidden) and introduce yourself to whomever you find there. I think of this as overcoming the barricades—think French Revolution—and meeting the enemy, who then quickly ceases to be an enemy. Start to interact with these people on a regular basis. Try a casual breakfast or lunch and then expand to social evenings with spouses. You will quickly stand out as a "go to" person on clinical matters, and you will also be privy to a great deal of information that your colleagues do not have. This makes you a valuable commodity to both administrators and trustees, both of whom will love the attention from a physician; and your physician colleagues will also be drawn to you for information that only you have. Everyone loves to gossip, and this is prevalent in the hospital setting so ignore those physicians who think you have gone over to the other side. Time spent with administrative leaders in your hospital will bring significant benefits to your daily activities as well as to your long-term career maturation. Try to speak with an administrator every day about substantive business in your hospital. Who knows—you might actually like the administrators. For me, developing real friendships with physicians and other clinicians has made my career infinitely more satisfying. I have learned much more about patient care than most administrators ever do, and this has allowed me to do a better job. My social life has also benefited—doctors' drink better wines at their parties!

By the way, don't forget to drop administrators' names into conversations with other doctors. Use only first names to show how close you are.

4

What Committees Should I Serve On and Why?

I know committee participation is one of the least desirable required activities for physicians. But guess what—most administrators do not enjoy attending committee meetings either. It is, simply put, part of the job for all of us, and a great deal of hospital business is conducted this way. The key question is this: which committees are worth your time?

Pay Me!

The Joint Commission and various regulatory bodies mandate many committees. These meetings must take place, and they often do contribute to the improvement of patient care or are needed for the normal functioning of the organization. Physicians must be present for these committee meetings to function efficiently, and the best way to assure physicians' presence is to pay them to attend. It is simply not fair to continually ask private physicians to take time away from their practices and not compensate them for revenues lost.

The Important Committees

In my view, physicians should try to involve themselves in four types of committees, whether paid to do so or not:

1. Any committee attended by members of the board of trustees

2. Any committee that reviews financial performance and makes monetary decisions

3. Any planning committee

4. The committee that makes capital project decisions

In practice, these four functions are likely to overlap and may not actually constitute four separate committees. Further, any committee making major decisions will likely have trustee membership, although some hospitals keep board committees and management committees distinct from each other. I do not advocate this, since I believe that trustees should get first-hand information about the hospital themselves rather than allow for filtering to take place by their administrators. The most important people to provide this information to the decision makers, as I advocate throughout this book, are the hospital's physicians. Management needs the input of physicians, and committees making decisions that affect patient care in any way should require that all clinical disciplines involved be represented.

> **For everyone: Stop bringing other work to meetings. There is no better way to label a meeting as unimportant.**

Getting a list of hospital committees and trustee committees, as well as their membership and meeting schedules, is usually simple. Your new best friends in the administration or medical staff office can help you with this. You must also learn when members are appointed to these committees and whether or not there are term limits. Some institutions do not impose routine term limits on committee membership, medical staff leadership positions, or even trustee terms. It is a generally held view that rotating new members into committees and leadership roles is beneficial to maintaining a fresh perspective on the business of the hospital and can also help bring new skills into the discussion as the needs of the organization change.

This information regarding schedules, purposes, and terms will allow you to determine what committees you wish to participate in and when new members are appointed and by whom. Since you will have already become close to the key leaders of the organization, it will be relatively straightforward to ascertain who must appoint you to the desired committee.

> **Physician tip: Make sure you introduce yourself to everyone on the committee.**

It is then up to you to participate in the business of the committee. This will likely require you to become knowledgeable regarding the business of the committee so that your input will be desired and respected. Becoming educated in the matters that come before the committee is your responsibility, and doing so will result in your becoming perceived as a leader. Few things are more frustrating than listening to someone pontificate about a topic he or she knows little about. Attend the meetings, make certain that you meet all the members, and offer useful information and opinions, and the return for your efforts will be worthwhile.

5

Working with Residents, Hospitalists, and Intensivists

This chapter is about some of the key people with whom physicians work in the hospital setting and with whom physicians share responsibility for patients. Obviously, physicians interact with many other professionals as well, particularly nurses; however, the parties discussed in this chapter have some degree of clinical decision-making authority regarding the care of the patients you admit to the hospital.

There are a few common themes regarding the needs of these three categories of physicians, even though the three types of physicians play very different roles in the hospital setting. Residents are there for postgraduate medical education in a specialty and are also hospital employees. Hospitalists and intensivists are hospital employees fulfilling a particular function. Hospitalists generally are focused exclusively on managing inpatient care and are supposed to be experts in that function. Intensivists are usually in place in the various intensive care units and are knowledgeable in the critical care provided in those units. In all cases, these individuals know more about how care is provided in their areas of responsibility, both in terms of the staff working there and the equipment and supplies available, due to their specialization in these functions. They may also have expertise in managing care through specific clinical pathways that are designed to provide optimal care and to move the patient through the system quickly and efficiently.

This is a particularly important discussion since these people play very specific roles in the hospital setting, often exercising authority over your patients while controlling assets and resources to which you want access. Physicians who want to work in the intensive care units are not happy to learn that this is not allowed in some hospitals that utilize intensivists. In fact, residents and hospitalists also will often exercise some level of authority and control over your patients. It is essential to understand the roles of these doctors and to develop useful and collegial relationships with them.

First, and most important, you should be available to them and should provide them the information you have gathered regarding your patients. The worst thing you can do in developing these relationships is not return a call. It is highly upsetting when a physician is unreachable for some period of time. No one, of course, is always available immediately, but you must make a good faith effort to be in communication when needed.

Second, you must acknowledge the mutuality of responsibility regarding your patients. You have admitted your patients to this hospital because you believe it is in their best interests. Hopefully, you have read this manual and are aware of how the hospital works, and nothing is going to surprise you. Therefore, it is incumbent upon you to work cooperatively with these colleagues. Nothing amazes me more than the physician who does not work willingly with these clinicians. They did not just appear from outer space!

Last, have a plan for the care of your patients after their hospital stays are over. One of the most frustrating situations in a hospital—and unfortunately, a very common situation—is for the patient to be unprepared to go home or to another institution. We all know this is something faced every day in every hospital, but to the extent possible, it is the responsibility of the attending physician to assist in the eventual placement of his or her patients. It is understood that many patients' post-hospital placement is often an insurmountable societal problem, but at least try to help. Ignoring the situation does not make it go away, and your reputation can only benefit from your attempt to be helpful.

Residents

One of the things that bring patients to the hospital is the twenty-four-hour coverage that hospitals provide. Nurses supply most of that coverage, but the residents, or house staff, play a critical role in allowing you to sleep through the night knowing that your patients are well cared for. All the residents want is for you to provide them some teaching in return for their services, particularly if there is something of interest in a patient's illness. Residents will also take care of your routine patients without complaint if you make yourself available to them for their education whenever you are there. This seems simple and straightforward, but you would be surprised by how often this does not happen.

> **Physician tip:** They know you were a resident once. Stop comparing the "old days" to their residencies.

Hospitalists

As a good friend of mine says, if you have seen one hospitalist program, you have seen one program. Each program is different, and each hospital with such a program in place defines the hospitalists' roles and responsibilities differently. Your first challenge is to find out how your particular hospital defines the position. Then take the time to sit with the hospitalist chief and work through how he or she will take care of your patient and determine what he or she needs from you. (This advice applies to everyone discussed in this chapter.) Commonly, a hospitalist will be your adviser and will not have the final say on a patient's plan of care, but some hospitals do give hospitalists the authority to make and implement decisions. If that is how a hospital operates, and you object to it, admit your patients elsewhere.

There is an increasing body of evidence that skilled, mature hospitalists can have some incremental benefit toward reducing lengths of stays and improving patient movement through the care process. Due to this, it is increasingly likely that you will see additional programs starting up, particularly at the more sophisticated hospitals. Determining how to work with these people will put you ahead.

Intensivists

These physicians are highly trained experts in place at most tertiary-care hospitals. These hospitals have determined that individuals who specialize in that critical care can best manage the complex and expensive resources available in the critical care unit. This is not surprising, since we know that any health-care service is best performed by people who perform that service often, and this applies to both hospitalists and intensivists. This is particularly true for the complex level of care provided by all intensive care units. In addition, this is also the most expensive care delivered in the hospital, and it is in everyone's interest to utilize these resources as efficiently as possible. Again, be available, communicate what you know about the patient, and be aware of what authority the intensivist has in caring for your patient.

To summarize, each of the parties to the transaction of patient care has differing needs, responsibilities, and skills. It is the blending together of each of these skill sets that makes our health-care system the envy of the entire world. When the blending is done correctly and with support from all the professionals involved, the patient and the system both benefit. The referring physician gets the best care for his or her patients as well as the twenty-four-hour supervision that is needed, all the professionals receive satisfaction from their chosen roles in the system, and the hospital and the health-care system strive to manage resources optimally.

Administrator tip: Don't start these intensivist and hospitalist programs without medical staff support and agreement.

PART II
Necessary Financial Knowledge

6

How Does the Hospital Make Money?

This is one of the more confusing areas of discussion regarding hospital practice. Much of the confusion is intentional, I believe, though a great deal of this lack of understanding results from the involvement of multiple parties with different agendas and perspectives. This includes the federal and state governments, legislatures, employers, insurance companies, and even individual hospitals themselves. All of these parties contribute to the bewildering state of hospital finance and, ultimately, to how hospitals make money.

Since my goal is to make complicated issues more readily understood, I will bypass lots of academic matters and cut to the chase. Simple rules can guide us here, even though the reimbursement regulations and insurance company guidelines are constantly changing, becoming ever more mysterious and illogical. Here are a few principles to understand to see how hospitals try to wring a profit from your patients.

> **Administrator tip: Everyone will appreciate a one-page summary of your financial results.**

Some Insurance Plans Are Better than Others

This is a widely understood rule of thumb and does not require much discussion. Depending on your locale and the roster of insurance programs available to your patients, both physicians and hospitals will make more or less money taking care of certain patients rather than others. This is not often an entirely controllable situation, usually due to geography, but all parties strive to have a so-called better payor mix (i.e., patients whose insurance pays more for the care provided). Hospitals watch for physicians whose patient populations contain better-paying patients and are very sensitive to physicians who admit one type of patient to a certain institution and a better-insured patient to another.

> **Physician tip: They will know if you are sending the good cases elsewhere.**

Surgical Patients Are Better than Medical Patients

In general, hospitals make more money from patients who undergo surgery. The procedures are usually reimbursed at a higher rate than is the care for a typical medical patient who generates only a daily room rate. Although both types of patients may produce a so-called case rate rather than a daily charge, the surgical patient's rate includes the operative procedure rate, generally a moneymaker. Now, though these are wild generalizations, they are accurate often enough to be used as rules of thumb. Yes, length of stay matters, as do many other issues, but the hospital that has more surgical patients than medical patients makes more money.

The More Procedures, the Better

Patients who undergo tests and procedures generate both technical and professional fees. The physician who oversees the test or reads the results of the procedure generally receives the professional fee, and the hospital usually receives the much larger technical portion of the fee. (This could be a separate generalization: technical fees are better than professional fees.) Physicians, many of who are building freestanding facilities designed to capture both portions of the fees paid, are more readily understanding this issue. For hospitals, this is a serious concern since they make a very large percentage of their money from these technical fees and are very reluctant to see them go or, heaven forbid, to share them with the physicians that generate the procedures. (Legally, of course—don't forget those pesky federal regulations.) Nevertheless, the more things that happen to the patient (tests, diagnostic or therapeutic procedures, or operations), the more money the hospital generally makes.

Shorter Stays Are Better than Longer Ones

This generalization is the result of all the focus on length of stay and the evolution of payment schemes that reward shorter stays and may even penalize the hospital for lengths of stay over the guideline for a particular diagnosis. The term for this is denied days, as mentioned earlier, and physicians who generate lots of them are on the wrong list when it comes to being valued by the institution. There is a target length of stay for every patient, and an incredible bureaucracy within the hospital attempts to manage the care of the patient to stay within this target. Be aware of this and know that patients who overstay their targets will require documentation from the attending physician as to why. Readily provide this information when asked and you will be a star!

Patients Need to Have a Place to Go When Their Care Is Over

A corollary to the previous rule is that some patients, often the underinsured and indigent, represent large potential money losses to the hospital, particularly if they do not have a place to go after their acute-care stay is completed. This next place may be their home or another type of facility, but regardless, the patients who linger in the hospital are costing the hospital money if their ongoing care needs do not justify their staying there; they are also likely blocking a bed from receiving a paying patient. It is not uncommon for a hospital to have a number of patients with stays of one hundred days or longer, the cost of which is generally not reimbursed. A savvy physician is armed with this knowledge and tries to assist the institution in finding the appropriate disposition for the at-issue patients. Again, hospital administrators know which physicians generate patients who are disposition problems, and at best, administrators do not look favorably on those physicians; at worst, they may actively seek to limit admission of those physicians' patients.

Complex Cases Are Better than Simple Ones

Many conditions that once were accepted for inpatient care are today assigned ambulatory or outpatient care status. Getting such inpatient stay approved takes a great deal of effort by the hospital staff as well as by the attending physician, and these efforts are likely to be viewed negatively.

Conversely, complicated cases, often those that require a surgical procedure, frequently result in a high case mix index (CMI). This statistic is a calculation of the severity of a patient's illness, and higher numbers result in increased payments to the hospital. It is easy to understand that sicker patients require more resources and that insurers pay more for the care of these patients. For example, organ-transplant patients and heart surgery patients are assigned some of the highest CMIs. The higher the CMI, the better the hospital's opportunity to make more money. Unfortunately, physicians do not automatically receive higher professional fees for these cases, something that has never passed the logic test for me since physicians must expend more time and effort to take care of sicker patients as well.

> **Physician tip: Let the administrators know that you understand this stuff.**

This is a greatly oversimplified discussion of how a hospital creates a profit. This discussion ignores the arcane and complicated formulas and algorithms that are actually used by insurers and third-party payors to determine how much money the hospital receives since this information is useless to the typical physician or manager on a daily basis. In fact, this is the type of information frequently used to confuse all parties. Nonetheless, these rules summarize the information needed by all parties to understand what is going on and how the hospital generates its bottom line. Hospitals whose policies and patient populations do not follow these models have a more difficult time making a profit and can often be in financial difficulty. Physicians and hospitals need to work together to take care of their patients within the constructs presented here so that all parties may have a harmonious relationship and a successful financial result.

7
Understanding the Operating Budget

The hospital operating budget is a lengthy, complex document that serves many purposes for varied audiences. It is often the closest thing to an annual operating plan for the organization that you will see, since the monies allocated for particular programs indicate the priorities for the institution for the coming budget year. The budget is also the vehicle for the board of trustees to approve the administration's plan for the year, and adherence to that budget is usually the major way in which the administration is held accountable for its performance. Failure to meet budget targets is one of the most common reasons for an executive to lose his or her job. (By the way, the most frequently cited reason for administrative turnover is the inability to get along with the medical staff—you would think this would motivate the administrators to work harder at developing productive relationships.)

The budget is also used by external bodies to monitor hospital performance. These entities, which may include banks, regulatory agencies, and bondholders, are interested in ascertaining what the hospital's plans are for the coming year, and they will also examine how closely the institution complies with these plans. A hospital management team's failure to be a good predictor of future performance is not indicative of superior performance.

> **Administrator tip: Involve key physicians in a meaningful way. They will know if you just want a rubber stamp.**

As you might expect, hospitals try to develop conservative plans that will accurately predict their upcoming performance. "Making the numbers" is everyone's goal, and having the right numbers in the plan is critical to the longevity of the management staff. Budgets, therefore, tend to be developed with significant wiggle room so that the targets can be met. That said, there are some major issues in the development of an annual operating budget that must be understood in order for a physician to have an impact on this activity.

Budget Realities

Most of the budget is committed before it is ever developed. For most, if not all, hospitals, roughly 60 percent of the operating budget is committed to wages and benefits for the hospital's workforce. The only major decisions to be made here are whether to grant pay increases to the workforce and whether there will be changes to benefits. Most institutions have some sort of cost-of-living increase, based on the local inflation rate, and they also may have market or merit increases. Market increases are usually the result of changes in the average wages paid in their region, sometimes for a particular profession like nursing. If shortages develop for a certain skill, the practitioners of that skill are able to demand an increase in compensation. It is also possible that union contracts mandate a certain increase for their members.

Merit increases are meant to reward and retain high performers and are very important for keeping the stars in your workforce from leaving for better wages at another hospital. Benefits such as medical insurance and pension plans also have to be evaluated each year so as to manage the cost to both the hospital and the employee, as well as to keep the benefit program current and up to the standards expected by the hospital's workforce.

Administrator tip: Physicians hate turnover of staff with whom they work. Don't lose people over relatively small amounts of money.

A well-managed organization has an effective program which includes an administrative staff that oversees wages and benefits and that takes all these matters into consideration so that the hospital retains the highly skilled and motivated workers it needs. Failure to do this results in unwanted turnover in key positions that will adversely affect the quality of patient care. Physicians are wise to keep an eye on turnover as an indicator of hospital performance.

After wage and benefit decisions are made, there are few matters left to the management team and the medical staff. If there is outstanding debt, as there almost always is, debt service payments must be made. Supplies and services like electricity and water are usually fairly predictable based on history and known price increases. Eventually most of the budget is committed and there are only a small number of ways that the budget is open to manipulation.

Institutional capacity drives revenues. Bed capacity and many outpatient services fix the number of patients that can be served. Obviously, no program operates at 100 percent capacity, but most have a utilization level that is accepted as efficient. For example, a program may work best when inpatient beds are at 85 percent occupancy, allowing sufficient capacity for emergency admissions, patient transfers, and staff performance. Higher occupancy may result in more frequent errors as well as staff dissatisfaction as stress levels increase. Moreover, some institutions are faced with contractual or regulatory mandates for certain professional staffing ratios and cannot deviate from them without penalty. The main point here is that it is difficult to increase revenue when services are operating at an efficient level. In these cases it is necessary to increase capacity or add new services to see revenue growth.

> **Physician tip: Make sure you know what you are talking about when you recommend a new program.**

Severity of illness is an important concept to understand. Most physicians are familiar with the previously described case mix index. This measure attaches a numerical value to each diagnosis and is used by Medicare and some other payors to reimburse the hospital for its inpatient services. Remember that the hospital makes more money if the case mix index climbs. Physicians who bring in more complex patients bring higher hospital revenues without increasing capacity.

Cash Is King

Though most of this discussion focuses on the operating statement, the balance sheet contains one item of importance to understand. The cash balance and the liquidity discussion are worth reading and understanding. Much of the financial jargon is confusing to the average person, but it is necessary to see that the institution is generating sufficient cash flow to take care of both operational needs and capital expenditures. Borrowing may commonly occur, but a successful institution borrows for major capital programs, not for its daily operational needs. If there is a line of credit being tapped for routine cash flow needs, something is out of balance. Take the time to review this matter and understand it since managing cash flow is essential to the overall success of the hospital (as well as your practice, your household, and so on). If you follow nothing else, follow the cash balance. Cash is king!

So What's Left?

It is well understood that hospitals have very small profit margins. In fact, many nonprofit hospitals in the United States lose money on health-care operations. There is constant pressure to shave costs and to have some net profit for reinvesting in the organization. There is much evidence that lowering costs, while often necessary, is only one piece of the puzzle. For a hospital to be successful, it must also generate new revenues, either by increasing the utilization of existing services or by developing new programs. For physicians and smart administrators, this is the area in budget development where the groups must interact.

In my experience, physicians are the most market-sensitive participants in the hospital environment. They most often know what new technologies are being developed, and they know what is going on in their fields of expertise as well as related ones. Whether it is by attending professional meetings or by visiting with salespeople in their offices, it is likely that they have more new program ideas than most administrators, and they need to be part of the budget-development process. Hospitals cannot save themselves to prosperity. They must expand their revenue base each year in order to generate the funds needed to reward their workforce and maintain their physical plant. Having a new program or business-development process in place that utilizes the expertise of the physician leadership is an absolutely essential part of a successful budget-management program. If this process is not in place at your hospital affiliation, the physician leadership must pursue its adoption. Hospitals that do not grow will automatically shrink as inflation and mandated expense increases eat away at existing revenue. Either you increase the size of the pie, or everyone gets a smaller piece.

8

Capital Equipment: Getting What You Need

Equipment acquisition is another key process for physicians to understand if they are to be successful in the hospital environment. All too often, physicians simply ask the hospital leadership for a piece of equipment and assume that because the item requested is the latest and greatest or because it will add a needed service to the hospital in its arms race with neighboring hospitals, the equipment will automatically be purchased. Invariably, this is an issue that leads to conflict among the parties and great dissatisfaction. It can even lead to losing a key physician to the competition.

In my view, both parties are to blame. The acquisition process needs to be transparent to all the players and needs to involve the input of all members of the hospital community. Frequently, the administration acts like it does not want the medical staff to know what the process is, who the decision makers are, and what the schedule is for making decisions and purchases. Conversely, physicians may simply ignore this information and make their requests when the mood strikes them. It is rather frustrating when a capital equipment request is made just a few weeks after the capital budget has closed for the year, particularly when all concerned agree that the equipment is needed. Although most institutions keep some dollars available for emergencies and unknown items, it may be a small amount and not enough for what is needed.

Administrator tip: Yes, chief medical officers are important, but include the physicians who actually use the equipment.

Understand the Process

The capital budgeting process, along with the operating budget process, usually happens on a semi-fixed schedule each year. Knowing the fiscal year dates is the first step, and asking to see the budget planning schedule, if it is not routinely published, allows the medical staff to understand when requests must be made. In a mature organization, there will be a strategic plan and a list of priorities or budget objectives published at the start of the planning process so that all parties can understand what the goals are for the organization for the coming year. In the absence of a plan or a set of goals, everyone is forced to make recommendations and decisions without a framework to assist them. (This is obviously not the best way to make decisions.) The hospital will also likely have an amount of money dedicated to the capital budget, and it is important to know what the amount is and how flexible it may be. To the medical staff, the source of these funds is less important than the amount available.

The hospital may also have a form or process to follow in evaluating a capital-equipment investment, and it is essential for the requesting party to utilize this methodology to help make its case. Although the equipment request is, hopefully, driven by concerns for quality of care as well as by financial concerns, the physician or the physician's practice administrator should be able to complete the analysis and have a good assessment regarding the viability of the request. For example, priorities are likely to include patient-safety items, replacement of out-of-date equipment, and facility repairs and replacements. Beyond those items, the hospital will often look then for new business and revenue opportunities, new markets to enter, and state-of-the-art "whiz bang" stuff designed to make a splash in the region the hospital serves. More often than not, the requesting party must calculate the return on investment for the piece of equipment as well as be able to address what other institutional priorities the equipment meets. This basic information makes your request stand out as prepared and thoughtful and separates you from the typical physician requestor. Further, the administration is not likely to ignore a request that adheres to the process and schedule. This information truly makes the administration's job easier and will be greatly appreciated.

Physician tip: Return on investment is a useful concept to keep in mind for all your business decisions.

Understand the Budget Drivers

What does this mean? Every hospital administrator thinks that every physician wants the latest piece of equipment for his or her use. But I would argue that it is better for all concerned to have available the newest technology, particularly when we all know how fast medical knowledge changes, and new equipment or devices are vast improvements. Moreover, the new item may even be required to correct a patient safety issue or to make certain that the institution is providing the expected community standard of care.

Utilizing the process described previously, physicians can go a long way toward understanding what is driving the budget thinking for their hospital. Being aware of priorities and understanding return on investment helps the decision makers in assembling a capital budget. It is also useful to look at past years' priorities to see where major investments have been made since it is common for the administration to want to be equitable and make investments in all service lines over time. For example, if a sizable chunk of the budget went to radiology over the past two years, it is likely that investments in other services are warranted and justifiable. On the other hand, it may be a waste of time to request something in an area that has been fully capitalized recently. Understanding what is behind the budget is essential to formulating a successful request.

Who Are the Decision Makers?

In every institution, the board of trustees must approve the budget. Some boards simply rubber-stamp the recommendations made to them by administration, and others are deeply involved in the actual decisions. It is important to know who actually makes the final decision regarding a capital investment and to make certain that this individual or group is fully informed about your request. A typical final budget request may be a brief summary of the item and its need and may lack some of the key information put into the original request. The person presenting the budget request also may be someone from a financial department who is unable to articulate the clinical rationale for the device, thus forcing the board to make a decision with incomplete information. Though I feel strongly that there must be clinical representation during both the budget formulation process and the actual presentation to the decision makers, certain hospitals keep the clinical leadership out of the process. Having invested a great deal of time and effort to formulate the request, the physician must be aware that the process is not over until the idea is sold to the decision-making body at the institution. Stay involved to the very end of the process, and you increase the potential for your request to be approved.

As is the case with everything else discussed in this manual, the prize in this situation goes to the most prepared. Understanding how decisions are made, when they are made, and who makes them will improve an individual physician's ability to influence the process and get what he or she needs for patients. Ignoring all of this and making a request at a random time, no matter your importance to the hospital, decreases the ability of the administration to make it happen and is as frustrating to them as it is to you.

PART III
Understanding the Institutional Environment

9

What Is a Health System, and Should I Care?

In theory, health systems were organized for two reasons: to organize and coordinate care across a region or community, and to allow for economies of scale and business efficiencies through larger entities having greater clout in the marketplace, especially in purchasing supplies and services.

Sounds simple and straightforward, right? Also sounds smart. These reasons for systems to exist would likely be true if health-care organizations acted like regular companies that operate throughout our economy (i.e., the people who work for companies do as they are told generally) and if hospitals delivered a product or service that could be easily replicated and centralized. Additional problems include the already discussed fact that the chief revenue makers, the physicians, do not all work for the hospital and the unfortunate truth that all too often, hospitals only join a system because they are failing financially, and they are looking for a bail-out. Though this may also be true when some for-profit companies merge, hospitals often fail because their core business, inpatient hospital care, loses money. Whether these losses occur because of inadequate reimbursement for care for high numbers of uninsured patients or because of an excessive number of competing hospitals in an area, joining a health system is unlikely to solve the problem. Frequently, a brief reprieve results when the health system improves some practices or even provides the struggling hospital with needed cash. But long term, the problems persist and require drastic actions, such as the pruning of low-demand or money-losing services or even the ultimate closure of the institution.

Administrator tip: System overhead does not produce revenue. No more fancy buildings—and get rid of that reserved parking spot.

At the core of many health systems is a very successful hospital, both clinically and financially, often the leading institution in its community. Someone in a leadership role at that hospital sees other area hospitals failing—often due to this hospital's own market dominance—and starts to think about saving these institutions. This thinking may be driven by ideas of developing a feeder network for certain services, maintaining an affiliated institution for some specialized activities, or keeping certain types of patients at those hospitals (usually the poorly reimbursed) or even by altruistically desiring to maintain jobs and dollars in the community. All of these reasons for developing a health system may make good business sense, and many systems have accomplished these goals and benefited their communities by doing so. Conversely, some health systems have failed miserably (see the Allegheny Health System in Pennsylvania, for example) and have even brought down or significantly damaged the core institution that financed the entire system. Most health systems are somewhere in the middle, having some modest success at coordinating care or achieving cost reductions through coordinated purchasing of supplies, equipment, or services or by development of new or expanded services for patients.

Unfortunately, though many academics have attempted to evaluate the success of health systems in accomplishing their stated goals, the answer to whether they have succeeded remains unclear. It is difficult to determine if the coordination of patient-care services has truly improved, if overall health-care costs have been reduced, or even if the rate of cost increase has slowed. Most likely, the definitive study has yet to be conducted and health-care systems are likely to continue to proliferate.

Impact on Physicians

Many physicians find their practices overrun by the development of health systems in their communities. The most frequent impact may be the opening or closing of a particular service, but a number of other events can impact physicians' practice of medicine as well. Such other possibilities include the following:

- The purchase of physician practices
- Changes in local hospital leadership
- Funneling of locally derived profits to the failing hospital
- The development of a costly system-overhead structure

- Pressures on physicians to change their referral patterns

This last issue may be the most important. System advocates commonly argue that efficiencies and improvements in the delivery of care will result from centralizing certain high-cost, complex services in one hospital location, and they urge physicians to send their patients to these centralized patient locations. Although this may be a good business practice, it may require physicians to disrupt long-standing referral patterns and personal relationships, delicately balanced interactions where patients move back and forth through an intricate network of relationships. Reasons cited for these referral patterns include history, geography, return referrals, and patient ease of access or perceived quality of the service. Breaking these referral networks is difficult to accomplish, and many physicians and administrators come to blows over this issue. The typical administrator overestimates the number of patients that may be diverted and often does not understand the personal and professional cost to the physician in disrupting the doctor's referral system. This results in physicians coming under intense pressure to make these changes. For all parties, the movement of patients to a new provider is a difficult element in ongoing interactions. Physicians must decide if they can confidently change their referral stream and not hurt their practices. This is a critical analytical process for a physician to deal with and cannot be done lightly or quickly. Physician colleagues within the practice or at other practices who have gone through this process can be helpful and may have a great deal of insight. External consultants may also be able to benefit the discussion. Helping the health system may be a positive action on the part of a physician, but harming one's practice in doing so is just plain dumb!

> **Physician tip:** Look for some of the signs that changes are coming—administrative turnover, late payments for supplies, shabby-looking landscaping.

In my view, the purchase of physician practices has proven to be one of the greatest failures of hospitals and health systems. Whether you subscribe to the opinion that physicians selling their practices do not work as hard as they did for themselves, or whether you hold the view that hospitals do not know how to manage the practices, the effort simply has not worked for the most part. Physicians who want to be full-time employees need to fully understand what that means, and hospitals can be more helpful in working through that process before the sale. In the long run, it is about more than money changing hands or assuming that because you own the practice, the patients will all come to your hospital.

It is not even certain that patients will stay with the practice. All in all, this is often a business activity that has not worked well for any of the parties and that requires a great deal more analysis and understanding before implementation.

A change in leadership is common when a hospital joins a system. This may happen overtly and in public, when the system replaces the hospital chief executive and some or all of the members of the board of trustees; or it may happen covertly, as the system moves the decision-making authority away from the hospital and up into the system. In some cases financial authority levels are changed since only the system leadership has the authority to make major dollar decisions.

It is important for each physician to understand where these decisions are now being made, what level of financial authority is assigned to each level of management, and even which members of the board are being retained. Physicians need to appreciate who is still helpful to them and who are the new decision makers with whom they must become acquainted. System development changes the power structure, and people may not have as much authority as they previously did in a freestanding institution. They may still be calling the same person "chief executive officer," but this does not mean that that person continues to exercise the same level of authority.

The last two possible impacts on physicians listed previously—the development of a costly system-overhead structure and pressures on physicians to change their referral patterns—are related, and both are controversial. Systems frequently move all member hospitals' profits and cash flows into the control of the system. Monies can be taken from the successful members of the health system to help subsidize the less successful organizations, and this may hamper a profitable hospital by preventing it from reinvesting earned resources toward its growth and development. This can be beneficial to the poor relations, but may ultimately slow down the growth of the leading hospital and actually hurt its market position. Over a long period of time, the entire system can flounder when the "cash cow" funding everything is no longer producing as much profit.

Last, physicians need to be on the alert regarding the development of corporate overhead. Many systems build new corporate offices, add staff, and increase salaries and benefits for system executives, sometimes paying system managers higher wages than the member hospitals' staff. Although it is important to manage and control the dollars being spent on these expenditures, it is also important to link expense increases to savings and infrastructure improvements. Additionally, some basic questions must be kept in mind: Does vacant space exist for corporate offices? Can certain hospital managers perform double duty as both hospital staff and system staff? Are any increases in the number of employees tied to new programs or direct savings? These and many other questions need to be answered, and physicians may be the only truly independent force left to hold the leadership accountable.

> **Administrator tip: Be prepared to explain why bigger is better.**

Health-system development can be very good for a community, by preserving jobs and improving patient care, but all parties need to be vigilant regarding how power and control are redistributed and where monies are being used relative to who generated those dollars. And it is most important to look for specific and demonstrable ways in which patient care is improved.

10

What Does a Trustee Do?

Many physicians I speak with ask about the board of trustees at their hospitals. Who are these people, what role do they play in the hospital, and how should physicians interact with them? These excellent questions, and many others, demonstrate the need for doctors to have more information regarding the people charged with overall responsibility for their institutions.

First, let me provide some background information about trustees. Whereas for-profit companies—and this includes hospitals that are for-profit—have boards of directors to oversee them, nonprofit hospitals are required to have a board of trustees to provide governance and leadership to all of the hospital's activities. The board's responsibilities include overseeing the financial health and stability of the organization, selecting the senior administrative leaders (including members of the board), and, most important, providing for the professional and administrative personnel, equipment, and facilities required to deliver safe and high-quality care to the hospital's patients. Trustees are responsible for performing these activities within all applicable licensure standards, relevant laws, and governmental regulations.

> **Physician tip:** Take the time to find out what the trustees do and why they want to be trustees.

Sarbanes-Oxley

A recent development in the for-profit world is the Sarbanes-Oxley legislation that details new standards for boards of directors regarding qualifications, conflicts of interest, and disclosure requirements, among other matters. Even though these regulations do not govern nonprofit organizations such as hospitals, many nonprofit hospitals have voluntarily adopted some of the prescribed standards, and many boards are evaluating whether to do so.

I find useful the Sarbanes-Oxley distinction between so-called inside versus outside directors and the legislation's limits on the numbers and percentages of each on a particular board. Applying this model to the charitable hospital setting, inside trustees would be members of the hospital management team, physicians who practice at the hospital, and anyone who receives some income from the institution. Outside trustees, required by Sarbanes-Oxley to be in the majority, are often community and religious leaders, volunteers, governmental officials, local business people, and political figures from the area served by the hospital. It is sometimes difficult to determine whether someone is an outside or inside trustee since a person who appears to be an outside trustee, perhaps a local business leader, may actually be receiving funds from the hospital through a business relationship his or her company has with the hospital organization. This is quite common in smaller communities where there is only one leading bank or law firm, and the hospital has little choice in whom to secure as a trustee or in where to receive needed services that are provided by the potential trustee's business. That said, these relationships must be described on a conflict-of-interest statement that every trustee should complete on an annual basis. These statements are public documents and may be viewed by an interested physician upon request.

> **Administrator tip: Trustees doing business with the hospital are inherently difficult. Be careful here!**

It should be noted that there is nothing inherently wrong with a trustee doing business with the hospital. As discussed, it may be difficult not to have some trustees with hospital business relationships on the board. These relationships must be disclosed, and the particular trustees must abstain from any discussions and votes affecting their businesses. In practice this is extremely difficult to monitor and some boards choose to simply not allow any business with companies affiliated with board members.

Trustees are rarely compensated for their efforts, aside from being reimbursed for expenses incurred in attending meetings. Most often, trustees perform their duties out of a desire to serve their community. In some cases, a personal medical issue has brought them to the hospital and given them a heightened sense of interest in the delivery of patient care.

It is here, in the delivery of safe and high-quality care, that the interaction between physicians and trustees becomes critically important to the achievement of the hospital's mission. Every hospital must have a formal structure in place for the organized medical staff to advise the board of trustees regarding the recruitment and retention of qualified and competent professional staff members (physicians, nurses, technical personnel, and so on), the selection of medical equipment, and the construction and maintenance of the hospital facilities. All of these matters come together to deliver the necessary patient care to the physician's patients.

The formal structure requires certain committees, such as a medical executive committee, a pharmacy and therapeutics committee, and others. These committees meet on a regular basis and have a membership of physicians, nurses, appropriate administrative personnel, and occasionally, trustees. In my view, the best-functioning committees include trustee membership so that the board of trustees may be advised directly by the clinical staff regarding matters of importance to patient care. When trustees are not present, information rises up to them through the normal filtering process of communication, and certain information may not make its way to the board. It is only human nature to try not to pass on bad news or to selectively provide information rather than disclose negative circumstances that reflect badly on individuals or hospital procedures.

In many hospitals, savvy trustees have their own informal mechanism for keeping tabs on the day-to-day operations of the hospital. Frequently, this starts with a medical need that brings them to a particular physician's office. That episode of care can blossom into a mutually beneficial relationship in which both parties share their knowledge and insight regarding the practice of medicine as well as the business of operating a health-care facility.

Failing the accidental connection, it is my advice that physicians seek out a relationship with a board member. Everyone benefits when the hospital's trustees are informed of key physicians' perceptions of the institution's goings-on without the filtering of hospital administrators. Obviously, it also allows the physician to press for a particular cause or service at the hospital or even for a new piece of equipment needed by the physician's patients. Though this may trouble some members of the hospital community, it is simply pragmatic for physicians to develop relationships with the leadership of their institutions. The delivery of health care is one of the most complex of human endeavors, and most trustees have only informal knowledge or experience regarding their organizations. It is, therefore, common sense that anything that increases trustees' knowledge will benefit patient care and make the trustees more effective board members. Conversely, the absence of useful, direct information can seriously impair the board's ability to successfully oversee the hospital.

In many states, regulations require that some or all board meetings be open to the public. Schedules of these meetings should be posted in the hospital and may be available on the hospital's Web site as well. Physicians are certainly welcome to attend the public meetings and become aware of the agenda that the board follows in conducting the hospital's business. It will become readily apparent that the majority of the matters considered relate to financial issues and that often patient-care issues may be discussed only briefly or not at all. This is where physicians can become actively involved in pursuing an agenda that places patient-care matters first. Engaged physicians make this happen, and it is both their right and their responsibility to get involved in the business of the board.

11

What Does Nonprofit Status Really Mean?

This is an area of hospital knowledge where jargon gets in the way of real understanding. This confusion results from the need of hospitals and health systems to meet technical requirements (i.e., those of the Internal Revenue Service Code) to be classified a nonprofit, charitable entity (commonly designated a 501-C-3 organization for the relevant section of the IRS code) while conducting business in a way that looks just like the business of for-profit companies.

Nonprofits make up the majority of our nation's hospitals and must meet various governmental regulations, which are primarily focused on the hospital's use of any profit for the benefit of the hospital. Confusing already, right? How can there be profit in a nonprofit? Some hospitals use euphemisms like "excess of revenues over expenses," but it is really profit. Bottom line: nonprofits hopefully have a profit; that profit just does not go to shareholders. They are also asked to provide some level of charitable care to the communities they serve. These two requirements—turning back any profit for use by the hospital and providing care to the uninsured and underinsured—are the key determinants of a hospital's nonprofit status. This is further complicated by the fact that the level of charitable care required is regulated in a confused manner by all levels of government, even the local townships, so that there exists no clear definition of how much free care is appropriate. Even the IRS has no definitive levels of charitable care and has provided little specific guidance.

Nonprofit hospitals perform all the tasks of any business—they build facilities, purchase equipment and supplies, pay salaries and benefits, and even merge with or purchase other hospitals. As noted previously, physicians and others often question why nonprofits can do some of the things they do, such as pay large salaries to certain executives, but they can conduct and do conduct all the business activities of any business. Clearly, the most controversial area today is that of salaries and bonuses for hospital leaders. High salaries were certainly not always the case, but recent years have seen an explosion in income levels as administrators have convinced many boards that their responsibilities equal those of executives in any business. Not everyone agrees obviously, and the IRS says one million dollars annually is too much, regardless of the size of the organization, but this area remains cloudy and is the cause of much disharmony in many hospitals.

> **Administrator tip: No physician will ever agree that you are underpaid. Now, overpaid—that's a different story.**

Though our country has urged hospitals to be more businesslike in their dealings, as a society we remain confused as to exactly how businesslike we mean. Using bill collectors to dun people who have no health insurance or charging whatever the market will bear for a service may be very businesslike, but it is certainly controversial. Stay tuned to this discussion; it is constantly in the news.

The most important benefits of nonprofit status are exemption from paying most taxes and the ability to utilize tax-exempt debt, thereby reducing the cost of borrowing money for capital items. It is exactly the coming together of nonprofit status and tax exemption that has caused the most concerns.

When both for-profit and nonprofit organizations conduct their business affairs in a similar fashion, governmental officials and political leaders begin to question why the nonprofit entities should receive a tax exemption. The most controversial issue appears to be hospitals using aggressive collection techniques for collecting past-due bills from uninsured patients. As a result of this, as well as because of concerns regarding high salaries, some localities have pressed hospitals to pay real estate taxes on the value of their land just like any other business situated there. Some members of Congress have held hearings addressing this matter, and a number of class action suits have been filed against some prominent nonprofit hospitals and health systems, questioning the health-care organizations' billing and collection procedures.

The bottom line: for-profit companies benefit their stockholders through the value of their shares of stock as well as through the distribution of dividends. Nonprofit hospitals turn back all money left after the payment of all expenses to the hospital for the benefit of the organization. After that, all hospitals seem to behave in a very similar fashion, and the significant increase in salaries for nonprofit executives, whether justified or not, has raised concerns at many levels of government and in many communities. Coupled with this, overly aggressive billing and collection practices have upset many as well. The long-held belief that a nonprofit, charitable organization meant lower salaries and a workforce dedicated to the mission of the hospital, while still operative for large numbers of people, has given way for some to a perception of well-paid staff and managers who install commonly held business practices and operate the hospital as a normal business entity. Though a famous mantra says, "no margin, no mission," this remains a situation begging for more clarity and agreement.

> **Physician tip: Whether nonprofit or for-profit, it still has to be run like a business.**

So what does this mean for the practicing physician? My advice is to not waste time and energy worrying about the technical differences between for-profit and nonprofit hospitals and health systems. Assume they all act the same regarding the patient-care process, all conduct their business practices in a similar fashion, and all hold their managers to the same high standards of performance. Whether they answer to shareholders or to the community they serve, in today's challenging business environment, they must all function with great effectiveness. If your hospital cannot convince you of its adherence to best practices and standards and does not meet your needs for taking care of your patients, find another hospital to practice at and do not worry about whether it is a for-profit or not!

PART IV
Topics of General Interest

12

Academic Practice versus Private Practice

At one time or another, almost every physician thinks about leaving academia for private practice or about giving up private practice to become a professor. No other profession has such a range of possibilities, and the ramifications of this career choice are dramatic. Since all physicians have had the first-hand experience of observing and participating in both environments, they are often better prepared to make this decision than they think. What is needed, however, is an objective review of the pros and cons of each option, relative to the personal and professional goals of the individual physician and his or her family. This chapter reviews the major points of this decision to help frame the discussion in broad strokes.

I should note for the record that it is my belief that academic medicine is where the majority of physicians secretly want to be. Observe the zeal physicians show in attempting to secure an academic appointment to put on their stationery. They may not want to expend the effort needed to meet the qualifications for a full-time appointment, but many are very happy to have a so-called prefixed or clinical appointment at a university to show their patients and colleagues.

Administrators Must Make a Choice Also

Physicians should understand that administrators must make this decision as well. Academic institutions are very different from community hospitals; specialty hospitals are different from general acute hospitals; and many people think that for-profit hospitals are different from nonprofit hospitals. Administrators must make important career choices and may not be able to move easily from one type of hospital to another. They get typecast fairly quickly as recruiters, and boards of trustees look for leaders with specific background and experience in their type of institution.

> **Physician tip:** You can try academic practice for a time without making a lifelong commitment.

Private Practice

The Pros. Depending on one's perspective, there are two significant positives to being in private practice. First, there is the potential for greater income. Every salary study I have ever seen shows that most physicians in private practice make more than their academic counterparts. Moreover, having worked in the academic environment for many years, I submit that it is clear that very few academic positions will provide greater income than private practice. Benefits may be better in the private sector as well, since physicians can tailor their benefits to their particular needs and may choose to devote a greater percentage of income to them. Leadership roles in academic institutions, such as department chairs or deans, may have sizable incomes attached to them, but these positions are rarely pursued for income alone.

The second major issue to understand regarding private practice is that of control. If you are running your own practice or are a partner in a group, you are likely to be much more in charge of your work and schedule than you would be in an employed status in the academic setting. Obviously, this is relative, since you may also be an employee of a physician group, but it is still probable that you will be able to exercise more control over your professional life and your personal time in the private sector. Mandatory hours, specific workloads, and committee participation are often mandated in both settings, but they always exist in academia.

The Cons. You are running a business in the private sector with all the attendant issues and problems. You are an employer having to select and retain qualified staff. You may have a building to maintain or at least a rental suite to keep clean and in proper repair. The cost of everything continues to go up. Malpractice is likely to be a major concern, but everything else you buy costs more each year as well, while the insurers who pay you may not increase your fees to keep pace with these rising costs. Physicians are often extremely successful as entrepreneurs, but many are not trained to make business decisions, and not every practice makes money. Some physicians find the competition for patients so intense in their fields that they simply do not bring in enough revenue. The list of potential issues and concerns in running a private practice rivals that of any business. More and more, physicians are opting for another option as these problems overwhelm them.

The Academic Life

The Pros. Academic life is different. The jobs are usually more varied in that patient-care duties make up only part of the job. Research and educational activities are ingredients in every academic physician's position, and this is what often brings physicians to these settings. Participating in the education of young practitioners is extraordinarily rewarding (my personal bias is showing), and being at the leading edge of medical practice is tremendously exciting. The prestige of being an academic physician, a professor, is highly desirable, and the interaction with students and researchers keeps one up to date and in touch with everything going on in the profession. Even popular literature reports that patients expect and presume that the best health care is delivered in the academic setting. This is where the action is.

The Cons. Income in academia is generally lower. It is pegged to regional and national standards reported by the American Association of Medical Colleges, and the information is readily available. It is essential that you research this information early on. No one can make the excuse that he or she cannot know what the salary range is likely to be for a particular specialty.

Control is generally less available. You may be assigned tasks relative to your academic rank that may not be to your liking, although you should be able to sort this out before you accept a position. Hours may be longer since you have more duties to perform or have to write papers or do research after your normal workday. In general, you may go from being the king of your own hill to being one of many princes in the kingdom. This is not necessarily a bad thing, but just different and requiring adjustments on your part. Academic institutions have bureaucratic structures to follow and limit advancement to people who understand how to fulfill the needs of the bureaucracy. Each school's approach to issues such as tenure or job security is likely to be different and should be studied thoroughly. Securing tenure requires a great deal of effort and may be beyond the grasp of some. Tenure itself is changing and may no longer mean lifelong financial security at many institutions. Some schools require a certain academic progression in rank and may deny an employee continued employment if he or she fails to achieve that progression. Hierarchies may be rigidly applied with chairs and deans exercising a great deal of oversight to your daily life.

The academic life can be extremely rewarding, but it is different from private practice and not for everyone. The worst mistake any physician can make in this situation is to expect that the field can be manipulated to be just like the private practice world. This is highly unlikely and will just result in a great deal of frustration. Physicians choosing the academic side of medicine must do so with realistic expectations of what their work life will be like. Conversely, private practice has its own set of rewards and may be the right place for you. The assessment of which is best for a particular physician requires a great deal of thought and analysis. If considered carefully, the career choice will be appropriate and rewarding.

> **Administrator tip:** Teaching hospitals are truly different from community hospitals. Academic physicians are different, as well, from their community counterparts and meeting their needs is a distinct administrative skill set.

13

What Do I Need to Know about Information Technology?

Information technology, electronic medical records, and the Internet are matters that physicians, hospital administrators, and patients discuss nearly every day. Our society has been undergoing a computer revolution for some years now, and every aspect of our culture is touched by it, especially the practice of medicine and the delivery of patient care. In no other segment of society has the computer brought so much frustration and failed promise. Multiple record systems vie for everyone's interest, personal data assistants (PDAs) are in everyone's hands, and patients now come to the office armed with computer search results regarding their condition or their suggestion for the correct drug regimen. The federal government is attempting to provide leadership here, and in 2005, President George W. Bush suggested a goal of determining and installing a universal medical record system in the United States within ten years. Without question, a unified strategy is required here for our health-care system to continue to be the world's model of success.

For most physicians' practices, this has translated into a debate over whether to implement an electronic medical record system now or wait, with the majority of practices deciding to wait. Concerns about the lack of any overall format, the costs associated with system purchase and implementation, and the reduced productivity that always accompanies the implementation of a new computer software system have led to a low adoption rate for physician practices. Notwithstanding this, physicians need to make some decisions about a few key areas.

Physicians need to be knowledgeable about three issues regarding information technology. First and foremost is the issue of medical errors. A growing body of evidence indicates that the use of information technology can be a major benefit in the reduction of medical errors in two ways. The computerization of a patient's specific health information, both in the physician practice and in the hospital, and the portability of that information have the potential to allow caregivers to have accurate and timely health information on their patients whenever they need it. This information may be on a card that the patient carries or even in a chip imbedded in the patient's upper arm. Nevertheless, we all hope that medical errors resulting from incorrect information, legibility problems inherent in handwritten orders, and the absence of information can be overcome in this fashion.

The other area thought to be of benefit in the reduction of errors is the use of decision-support technology and clinical pathways. It is expected that physicians with access to these will be able to combine their personal knowledge and experience with the ability of the computer software to obtain full and complete knowledge of the appropriate plan of care for patients. Combining the physician, it is thought, with the computer program will further reduce errors as well as speed up care and possibly even reduce length of stay. Though some of these hoped-for results are not yet fully realized, there are some early studies showing that highly computerized hospitals that use these tools are showing lower mortality rates than their less computerized peers. There is much more work to be done here, but with the ever-increasing amount of medical information available as well as the inability of paper-driven patient-information systems to keep up, it is encouraging to see some of the progress being made here.

A second area of interest is that of using technology to improve productivity and reduce costs in the health-care delivery system. Many industries have been utilizing information technology for decades to improve the efficiency of their manufacturing systems, cost controls, inventory-reduction systems, and labor-utilization methodologies. In fact, most segments of our economy have made great use of computers in improving their results while health care has been lagging far behind. There have been many reasons (excuses) as to why this is so, including the complexity and lack of standardization of health-care services, the combination of art and science in the provision of care, and the unwillingness of some health-care practitioners to adopt computerized systems. Some practitioners still do not feel comfortable at a keyboard. Though these are real concerns, several leading institutions are showing the benefit of using information systems throughout the hospital, and there is a great deal more to learn and adopt, in administrative improvements as well as in patient-care delivery.

> **Note to all:** It makes sense to just install a basic electronic medical record system. Standardization will come later.

The last area of the three areas of interest is the rise of consumerism and the Internet. At no other time in the history of medicine has it been possible for patients to come into a discussion with their physician armed with as much information as, and sometimes more information than, the practitioner has. Studies show that as many as 85 percent of patients with the time and resources are becoming extremely knowledgeable about their health status, and they desire to become partners with their caregivers. Some physicians find this beneficial and useful in working with their patients; others consider it an intrusion into the physician's role. Using the Internet to gather information and communicate with their caregivers is a practice many people have adopted and use on a regular basis. Moreover, these patients expect to be able to communicate with the physician whenever desired and to receive a response on a timely basis.

Implications for the Physician

Every hospital needs to adopt an electronic medical record system and a management information system. The market includes many competing systems, just as many physician office systems are available as well. There is hardly a consensus as to what system is best, and there has been tremendous change in the marketplace, with companies entering and leaving the market frequently. The Centers for Medicare and Medicaid Services (CMS) has now entered the fray with the offer of a free software package for physicians' offices, although the practices have to pay the costs of installation and maintenance. This is the first time a government agency has, in effect, indicated a favorite system, and this may well serve to clarify some direction for the future, although it is much too early to see if a significant number of practices will take CMS up on its offer. Further, with the formation of a national committee to oversee health-care information technology policy, government is asserting an ever-larger role in the decision-making process. In any event, each practice needs to make a decision as to whether to adopt a system now, if it has not already, or wait to see who will survive in the marketplace.

Ultimately, the physician's office system, the physician's PDA, and the hospital's electronic medical records must interface smoothly with an individual's personal health-record system. Will we get there? Yes! When? No one knows, but make your decisions within this context. More time and money has been wasted on faulty IT decisions than any of us would like to acknowledge.

Physician tip: If you have not learned how to type, do it now! Dependable voice recognition is not happening anytime soon.

Practices must also address their use of the Internet and develop a Web site and an e-mail policy and system. Many patients seek out a new physician through the Internet, and most practices use their hospital or health-system affiliation as their method to be represented on the Web. If your practice is not doing this now, you can either seek out such an affiliation or start your own Web site. The latter is a costly and time-consuming activity and may not be economical for a small practice; however, it can be the source of a real market advantage when adopted. If you use your hospital's physician directory, it is smart to periodically check and see what information is being provided to the public. There can be significant errors and omissions, or it just can be out of date.

The use of e-mail is the last matter for consideration. If it is used to communicate with patients, a clear policy must be developed that defines how it is used and for what information. It may also be used to request or schedule appointments, allowing a practice an advantage over competitors that keep people on the phone for lengthy periods of time.

Physicians need to decide what their policies are here and communicate those policies to their patients. For example, do you personally respond to patient e-mails? Do you allow clinical questions? What other uses are allowed? Whatever you choose, it is essential to assign someone responsibility for the e-mail and Web site, to keep information on the Web site up to date, and to respond to patient e-mails promptly. If these practices are poorly handled, it will infuriate patients. If they are handled well, use of the Internet can give you a competitive advantage.

For a physician practice to survive and grow into the future, the physician and administrative leadership must become knowledgeable about information technology or at least make certain that this expertise is available to them. Today's marketplace, while diffuse and undirected, will eventually give way to some clearer direction as major health systems and government agencies determine a course of action. The significant benefits in improving care and increasing efficiency in the health-care delivery system are too enormous to be overlooked for much longer. Physicians need to be ready.

A word here about advertising and marketing: Most of us wonder why so much money is spent here and how much actually brings a measurable return. With so many studies showing how much the Internet is used by consumers in gathering information about every facet of life, including health care, physicians must make a conscious decision as to what type of Internet presence they wish to have. Moreover, in my view, if you do nothing else, spend the time and effort to make certain your Internet presence is that which you desire. I can't tell you that money spent on general advertising or marketing will achieve your goals, but I can assure you that money spent on an Internet site will yield significant benefits. Also, if you let your hospital be your "advertiser" here, make sure you are happy with what they are saying about you.

14

Hospital-Physician Integration: Making a Deal

Making deals is on the minds of physicians and administrators every day. This phrase—"making deals"—has become shorthand, maybe even code, for administrators' building relationships with the physicians who admit patients to their hospital. Administrators are trying to secure more business for their institutions, and physicians are worried about practice incomes falling and expenses rising, and they need to find ways to compensate for that. Both parties are convinced that insurers and government are out to reduce their expenditures for health care, and our entire society is worried about rising health-care costs. For many, making some sort of deal is the way to solve these problems. In fact, some physicians feel that making a deal with a hospital is the only way out of their particular financial problems.

Unfortunately, the government has a lot to say these days regarding how physicians and hospitals work together. The stated concern is that of illegal inducement—that is, anything that causes a physician to admit more patients to one hospital or to increase utilization of a service at a particular hospital. The watchdogs, using the Stark regulations, are out to make sure that no monies change hands to change utilization patterns, and there are many reasons for this legitimate concern. Studies have suggested that physicians have, in fact, over-utilized services when they have had a financial interest. As a result, numerous regulators now scrutinize and evaluate contractual relationships between doctors and hospitals. In addition, an equally large number of lawyers are ready to advise and structure these deals so that they pass all regulatory tests.

What Does the Hospital Want?

First, let's look at things from the hospital executives' point of view. The drivers of the hospital's revenues, the medical staff, usually are not employees of the hospital. In many areas, these physicians often work at more than one hospital. These so-called splitters come and go as they wish and admit their patients wherever they choose. For any manager, not having control over the means of production of revenue is a major concern.

No matter what your hospital administrators tell you, this fact of life drives them crazy. Every day they are thinking of ways to control your practice and get more business for their facility. The jargon used for this process is physician-hospital integration or, simply put, deal making.

The Possibilities Defined

This integration comes in many guises: paid medical directorships, contractual agreements for specific services, co-management deals, and other arrangements. Prior to the federal government's interest in limiting these agreements (Stark amendments, Safe Harbors), there was a never-ending list of possible perks, but the previously noted regulations have truncated the possibilities. The major concern in any relationships between hospitals and physicians is that they not have any element that suggests greater compensation for higher numbers of patient referrals. Beyond that, there are many potential pitfalls, and this is a major area in which both parties can get into trouble. A lawyer specializing in these arrangements is crucial, but keep in mind that anything that links compensation to utilization is unacceptable.

What Is the Goal?

The point here is not to suggest that these types of arrangements are necessarily bad or harmful to physicians or their patients. But it is important to craft them in a mutually beneficial way through understanding the administrators' true goals. Understand your leverage: increased admissions or procedures, needed attendance at medical staff meetings, and perhaps supervision of a unit or service. With this information in hand, the physician can make a deal that benefits all parties. Most important, beyond the legal construct, is that the arrangement be something that you want to do. Though it seems self-evident, don't agree to do something that you are really not interested in doing. Keep in mind your goals for your hospital practice and make certain that the activity furthers them.

Physician tip: It's just business, not personal.

For example, the hospital needs you to attend certain meetings, probably the most unpleasant thing on many physicians' lists of unpleasant things. Your attendance is likely to be an accreditation or licensure requirement. Most often, attendance for these meetings is small in numbers, causing major headaches for the hospital. There is nothing wrong with a physician requesting a meeting fee as compensation for time away from their practice. All parties win here, since attendance goes up, the committee's business gets the valuable input needed from physicians, and the patient-care process benefits. The accrediting entities are happy, and a major problem for the hospital is solved.

By the way, you only get the meeting fee if you show up!

Do You Want to Be an Employee?

At the other end of the spectrum of hospital-physician relationships are full-time employed positions, something increasingly of interest to many physicians. As practice costs rapidly increase, with insurance reimbursements not keeping pace and malpractice insurance costs getting wildly out of control, the idea of a salary can appear very attractive. Moreover, changing views of the physician lifestyle also cause some to look fondly on being an employee and getting home to dinner with their families more frequently. Very often, the hospital agrees with this view and a good deal for all can be made. Make certain this is what you want, or try to include an "out" clause in the transaction. (Again, this may be common sense, but physicians frequently make better self-employed businesspeople than they do employees.) It may not be easy to go back to your previous life, but don't assume anything. Put it in your agreement.

How to Make a Deal

This is not an in-depth discussion of how to make a deal, but some basic advice should be helpful:

1. Get an experienced advisor. The hospital exec has more knowledge and experience and has likely made many similar deals. Being a success in medicine does not mean that you know how to negotiate as well as your average administrator.

2. Be aware that the hospital is focused on achieving specific goals and wants to link incentives to these goals. Though this must be carefully constructed within existing laws and regulations, the hospital can be very specific in listing the exact behaviors they wish to elicit from you as long as they do not

indicate a relationship dependent on increased activity or admissions. These performance criteria can provide you a direct benefit in that achieving them results in greater income. These objectives can legally be directed toward achieving increased quality of care and patient-satisfaction goals. Stay away from anything that ties increased patient referrals or procedures volumes to increasing your income. This seems pretty simple, but questionable or illegal deals get made all the time. Also stay away from anything that involves partial ownership of an activity unless you are absolutely certain that you are not self-referring to that entity. All of this should be clearly understood and any suspect activity avoided.

3. Perhaps I mentioned this already—get help from an advisor who has negotiated these deals many times! I know you are a brilliant neurosurgeon, but you do not get to use a scalpel in this transaction—hopefully not, anyway.

Remember…

Having a business arrangement with the hospital can prove invaluable. It also can be a major problem. Although the added income may be helpful, make certain the activity you agree to perform is something you enjoy and really want to do. Money alone will never really motivate you to do something you hate. Moreover, taking money for something you do not intend to do fully and completely is just wrong.

> **Administrator tip:** You do not have to win every negotiation. All parties should walk away feeling good about the deal.

15

Oh, No! Not Another Quality Improvement Program

In the last thirty years, no area of hospital practice has received more attention than quality improvement programs (QIPs). Just inventorying the different types of programs tried and abandoned during this time frame would be a daunting task. Government at all levels, business associations, and health-care practitioners themselves have advocated for programs just to see them go away and be replaced with another. Sadly, as recently reported by the Institute of Medicine, medical errors remain a major concern, and the area of quality improvement continues to be a serious national problem. Moreover, a study published in the *Journal of the American Medical Association* in June 2005 reported what many of us already suspected. Despite billions of dollars spent, organized quality improvement programs show little real and lasting impact.

Why is this the case? Why does health care, unlike, say, automobile assembly, resist structured process improvement? I do not pretend to have the definitive answer, but my experiences have certainly provided some clues.

The first, and perhaps the most important, factor in my view is the failure of organized medicine to evaluate and adopt a particular methodology and promote its use. Such practices as evidence-based medicine and clinical pathways have many adherents and are in wide use, but neither of these appears to provide the total answer to quality and process improvement, particularly in the complex environment of the hospital.

Regardless of whether an optimal methodology currently exists, the best clue to the failure of QIPs is this lack of physician leadership. With no major physician group leading the way, QIPs have been left to administrators, business coalitions, insurers, and regulators. None of these groups has the clinical knowledge to either develop these programs or actually make them happen in the delivery of care. We must recognize that physicians and other clinicians are the ones who actually take care of patients, and they are the ones who will either adopt or ignore a QIP. It is a central tenet of change management that for people to actually support making changes, they must be deeply involved in the conceptualization and design of the change. Moreover, without physician and nursing leadership of the process, administrators and bureaucrats are simply unable to implement significant change on the hospital unit. In addition, administrative turnover and legislative changes cause many of these programs to be changed or dropped just as some positive results are occurring. Indeed, the Institute of Medicine has suggested that it requires seventeen years for major changes to the patient-care process to be adopted and actually become common practice. No particular QIP has yet been in place for any time period of this length, not even close.

Administrative turnover is a major issue when the hospital executive or the chief medical officer is the champion of the program. Frequently, just as a program is showing a useful result, one of these key leaders leaves the institution. The issue of changing legislative mandates is also a common problem with both state and federal programs being introduced on a regular basis without funding streams attached and with little physician leadership in their development.

Clearly, it is the responsibility of organized medicine and individual physicians to take charge of these efforts, or we will likely continue to lurch from program to program and not achieve the results we desire. This "flavor of the month" approach simply has not worked.

So what should be the posture of the individual physician or practice when approached by the administration to participate in a quality improvement effort? Simple: take charge of the program!

In the absence of medical leadership, QIPs have little chance of succeeding. Led by physicians who are true champions of quality improvement, programs are more likely to take root in the institutional setting. This seems so clear to me that I constantly wonder why there is not more organized physician leadership in this matter.

Physician tip: Patient care is your responsibility. Period.

Pay for Performance and Gain-Sharing

There is another aspect to quality and process improvement programs that is proving to be very controversial: that of employing financial incentives to motivate physicians to participate. Hospital executives are always looking for ways to partner with their medical staff members, but aligning the desire to improve care or reduce costs with money incentives has an unsatisfactory history. One only needs to remember when many health maintenance organizations provided bonuses to physicians for reducing specialty referrals or numbers of expensive diagnostic tests to see how the public, as well as legislative bodies, feel about this. Although discussion regarding pay for performance and gain sharing is widespread, physicians are advised to be cautious in participating in these programs. Patients must not feel that their care providers are conflicted in making judgments regarding their health-care needs, but rather must feel that physicians are willing and able to do what is best for them. Moreover, there is something wrong about letting the public think that physicians will only do what's right when they are paid to do so.

> **Administrator tip: Stop tying monetary incentives to quality improvement programs. Patients hate it!**

We all agree that delivery of the highest quality health-care services is our goal. Long lists of programs have been attempted with little lasting effect and a great deal of wasted effort and money. It is the responsibility of organized medicine and individual physicians to take charge of this aspect of health care and provide the leadership needed to determine the correct path to take. Even though there is a great deal of emphasis on providing financial incentives to physicians to participate in these programs, physicians need to be cautious about doing anything that may cause patients to question their motives. The physician-patient relationship, under fire for many years, needs to be foremost in the minds of caregivers.

It is also worth noting the so-called Hawthorne effect. Simply put, this effect is a management concept first noted in the early 1900s. Management researchers in a manufacturing plant saw that any attention paid to workers caused all participants to more carefully perform their activities, and the process almost automatically became more efficient. Conversely, when attention was taken away from the process, performance fell back to previous levels. The Hawthorne effect has been evident in health care for many years. Quality improvement programs always cause some improvement when they focus on a particular area. Unfortunately, the same reversion to previous levels of performance takes place in health care as well. For us to make any lasting improvement, we must be unwavering in our commitment. To date, this has not happened except in isolated institutions where true physician champions exist. We need more of them!

16

A Practical and Strategic Evaluation of Your Practice

A little bit of philosophy is necessary here before entering the heart of the discussion regarding the evaluation of practices. This discussion is not about selling your practice. Accountants and consultants can help you with that if you wish, but my personal opinion is that too many practices are sold to hospitals and others for the wrong reasons. The sale of a practice should come about for a relatively short list of reasons, including financial exigency or retirement, and the latter reason for selling can be prevented by bringing in an associate in the years prior to retirement. Financial exigency usually results from escalating expenses, especially malpractice coverage, or a significant change in payor mix. Other issues can cause this financial trouble as well, including facility or equipment needs, but these matters should not come as a surprise. These problems should be foreseen by the physician or the practice's management staff.

To me, the sale of a practice is a last resort and has proven not to be of long-term benefit to either the purchaser or the seller. Certainly, some physicians have benefited by selling off the practice and starting another when their noncompete agreements expire, and some have even been given back the practice when the purchaser, often the local hospital, has failed to accomplish the results they thought would occur with the purchase of the practice, usually increased admissions to the hospital.

In any event, before reading this chapter, you should be sure to read chapter 6, which discusses how a hospital makes money. Our goal here is to strategically evaluate your practice, not value it as a candidate for purchase by the hospital; this will help physicians and practice administrators determine the leverage they have in their dealings with hospital management teams. I am also striving here to provide administrators with a construct for understanding the value of a particular practice's patients to their institutions. Keep in mind that the common wisdom among administrators is that physicians greatly overvalue what they bring to the hospital, so the key here for physicians is having the data to back up any statements regarding practice value. Many administrators simply divide by half whatever the physician says is coming.

It should be noted again that the valuation of a practice for sale or purchase is a financial activity, and companies that specialize in this activity have the knowledge necessary for this process. If sale is your desired goal, consult one of these experts; however, the principles discussed here should affect the financial assessment and will best be accomplished first. A sound understanding of the strategic value of a physician's practice will increase the financial value for all the transaction's parties.

> **Physician tip: Your practice is about much more than money.**

The rules described in chapter 6 form the basis for a strategic evaluation. Most practices can easily quantify the number of patients they are seeing, particularly when they are in receipt of summary information from each insurer they deal with. Request this information from the insurers, but ask them to also tell you how many procedures, tests, and operations your patient population has generated. Some insurers will have this information, and some will not. Some will refuse to share it, which then requires estimates to be made by the practice administrator and the physicians involved. Real data is always best, but most physicians can estimate the hospital procedures that their patients require.

The real trick here is to translate the volume of procedures into an estimate of the patient and technical revenue this amounts to for the hospital. For example, if your practice generated 100 cardiac catheterizations per year for the institution, and the average technical revenue generated is $1,000 per procedure, then $100,000 in hospital revenue resulted from these referrals. Taking stock of every patient day and every procedure you provide to a particular hospital allows the practice's real dollar value to be calculated. This is a process not often undertaken since the information is difficult to collect, but this is worth doing before you bring in the accountants or consultants, or before you engage in discussions with the hospital. A sharp practice administrator, using the resources of the Internet, can put together this analysis and provide the practice leadership with a useful frame of reference of the dollars the practice generates for the hospital. Payment levels for each procedure from each insurer, both public and private, are available with some effort through state insurance departments and from the federal government for Medicare.

Another key factor in the discussion is your referral patterns. Where do your patients come from and what are their demographics (geography, insurers, income level, and so on)? Do other physicians refer patients to you, and if so, who are they and what are their relationships to your hospital and to others? What is the degree of influence you might exercise over these physicians? This is the type of information, coupled with the dollar impact of your practice that resonates with administrators and determines the strategic positioning of your practice for them.

Take note that a competent hospital executive will have this information and will have already put together his or her own assessment of what each practice is worth to the hospital as well. We are trying to level the playing field here.

So how do we use this information? Let's answer this by looking at a role-playing example using two approaches, the typical physician's approach to discussing a need with a hospital executive and my suggested approach.

For this example, let's suppose that a physician wishes to exert some influence on a hospital matter that will affect his or her patients. This could be a decision regarding a facility construction matter. The physician schedules a meeting with the appropriate hospital executive to push forward a specific viewpoint regarding this construction decision.

Traditional Approach

Physician: Mr. Jones, you know that I have been a loyal admitter to this hospital, and I want you to consider the needs of my patients in the new facility you are working on. I know I bring a lot of patients to the hospital, and it is worth your time to discuss this.

Administrator: Doctor Smith, I will absolutely include your thoughts in the analysis. Your opinion, and that of all the medical leadership, is very important to my colleagues and me.

(I have used this answer many times myself. It's a great answer that never fails to pacify some people, but it is obviously short on specifics.)

Administrator tip: Share the needed information if physicians ask you. It's about their patients.

My Suggested Approach

Physician: Mr. Jones, as you know, I bring a significant amount of business to this hospital. In fact, my practice administrator, who tracks this for me on a daily basis, tells me that we had more than XXX admissions here last year and that these admissions generated hundreds of tests and procedures. Our calculations show that our practice brings you over $XX million dollars of revenue annually and that we are growing at a 10 percent rate each year. Let me show you the financial pro forma we have developed regarding this as well as the information we have gathered to confirm the numbers. This makes us one of the five largest practices at the hospital and leads me to ask you for a role in the decision-making process regarding our new facility.

I also want to show you where my patients come from and what physicians refer to me and give you a sense of the strategic value of my practice to the hospital.

Administrator: Wow! Let's go over your data. I am really impressed that you have prepared this information. Then we can discuss what you want.

Simplistic? Of course. Does it happen often? No, but that is my point, and the likelihood of physicians being involved in key decisions rises with the amount of hard data they bring to the table.

The typical unprepared approach makes it easy for the administrator to brush off the medical staff, but real dollars on the table, with whatever implications might be drawn from this (never threats!), help focus the hospital's leadership on the real value of that physician.

This is the type of discussion that can be meaningful and useful for the physician and his or her practice. Understanding the strategic value of your practice is the most valuable knowledge you can possess in getting what you want and in becoming a key member of the hospital's team. Once you arrive at this status, you can expect to be consulted frequently about hospital decisions and can solidify and greatly increase your influence in the institution.

Part V
Closing Thoughts

Hospitals come in different flavors. Successful organizations just feel right. Nurses, doctors, and administrators work together easily and without being coerced to do so, high-quality patient care happens every day, and no one needs to organize meetings to tell people to do a good job because they just do it. The hospital atmosphere is positive, cheerful, and energized.

Conversely, poor hospitals are easy to spot as well. No one gets along, the leadership is constantly nagging staff to do better work, the hospital is negatively charged, and you just get a bad feeling walking into the place. These facilities often look dark and dirty, and it just seems that no one cares. Not surprisingly, these facilities often have poor malpractice records, and many physicians understand that poor quality hospitals can impact their own malpractice status since they may be named in lawsuits in which the hospital staff is at fault.

Very often, these negative characteristics result from the poor quality of interaction between physicians and administrators. The high-functioning hospital has mastered the art of having everyone work together, and everybody knows it. At one point in my career, I thought this was a reflection of size—the larger the hospital, the more difficult it is to manage. And though there is some truth to this, size can be overcome, and even the largest hospital can work smoothly. Smooth functioning requires that the key players be comfortable with each other and have the knowledge necessary to get the job done, provide the necessary staff, supplies, equipment, and facilities, and have all this come together on a daily basis.

Improving communication between parties is the idea behind this manual, and it is my hope that this small contribution will move physicians and administrators closer together. Although hospitals do not easily lend themselves to standardization due to the great complexity of the patient-care process, communication and credibility can be a standard applied to all parties. Increasing physician and administrator understanding of the daily life of the hospital from each other's standpoint has the potential to improve performance, increase satisfaction for all parties, and, I believe, even make the bottom line better. Hospitals that work more efficiently are better in every way, and this is what we all desire.

I would be remiss not to also add that I believe strongly that physicians are not doing enough to provide leadership to the health-care delivery system, either individually or on an organized basis. Recent articles about physicians profiting from legal, if not entirely ethical, schemes in processing laboratory tests reinforce my opinion. These stories came after previous reports of physicians overutilizing many services where they had an ownership stake or an investment. Though it is clear that a small minority of physicians are involved in these activities, it is incumbent upon all physicians to speak out against them, and their professional organizations must condemn them as well. Until physicians are able to restore their reputations as trustworthy and reliable stewards of patient care and take charge of the delivery of that care, their credibility with the public will not improve. Programs like gain sharing, though perhaps well intended, allow patients to question why physicians must receive some additional monetary reward for providing quality care. Linking all these matters together does nothing to enhance the status of the medical profession and will likely do little to improve care or reduce costs.

Physicians must be seen as the patient's advocate and must take control of the health-care system if we are to truly improve the quality of care.

A tip for all of us: If you have not been a patient lately, remember that it is not fun. In everything we do, we need to keep the patients in mind.

Appendix

Glossary of Terms

Academic Medical Center: An organization that includes, at minimum, a medical school and a hospital. There may be more than one hospital, and the medical school may be part of a larger college or university.

Accreditation: Determination by the Joint Commission on Accreditation of Healthcare Organizations that an eligible health-care organization complies with the applicable Joint Commission standards of care. The main focus of the standards relates to the safety and quality of patient care.

Capital Budget: The monies devoted to the purchase of equipment, furniture, and facility renovation and construction. Usually a fixed amount determined by the institution on an annual basis.

Case Mix Index (CMI): The accepted measure of the severity of illness for a given hospitalized patient, relative to the consumption of resources for that patient's care. It is displayed as a number in the format of 1.00 and higher. The hospital receives greater reimbursement as the number increases.

Chief Medical Officer (CMO): Usually a hospital employee, the chief medical officer is responsible to the chief executive officer for the delivery of care at the hospital.

Conflict of Interest: The determination that an outside business, professional, or contractual relationship on the part of a hospital decision maker may affect the judgment of that person. The organization must be aware of these relationships and take steps to make certain that decisions are made in the best interest of the organization.

Director: A legal term to identify a person who has the fiduciary responsibility to oversee the operations of a for-profit company and who is responsible to the shareholders of that entity, who as a group are known as the board of directors.

For-Profit Organization: An organization or company that shares profits with the owners or shareholders of the entity and pays taxes on its profits.

Gain-Sharing: See Pay for Performance.

Hawthorne Effect: This refers to the improvements in productivity or quality that result from extra attention paid to workers, rather than to actual improvements in methodology or process.

Health System: Usually made up of two or more hospitals or health-care organizations. The health system may have a separate corporate entity and leadership in addition to the leadership of the hospital members of the system.

Hospitalist: A physician who devotes his or her entire practice to the care of hospitalized patients.

Intensivist: A physician who devotes his or her practice to the care of patients in a specific type of hospital intensive care unit, such as a coronary care unit or a surgical intensive care unit.

Joint Commission on Accreditation of Healthcare Organizations (JCAHO): The Joint Commission is an independent, nonprofit organization established more than fifty years ago to verify and improve the quality of care delivered by hospitals and other health-care organizations through detailed, on-site surveys of the organizations. The JCAHO has an extensive set of standards of care that hospitals must adhere to in order to be accredited.

Medical Staff Bylaws: A governance framework for the organized medical staff of a hospital that delineates the roles and responsibilities of the medical staff in the delivery of care to their patients.

Nonprofit Organization: Under IRS guidelines, an organization that returns all profits to the organization for its continued development. No individual may receive any portion of the profits, nor does the organization pay taxes on its profits.

Operating Budget: The annual budget plan of a hospital that forecasts and manages the costs related to the staff, supplies, and expenses needed to operate the hospital.

Pay for Performance: Refers to a program that rewards physicians with additional income in return for implementing specific quality-of-care measures designed to improve the delivery and safety of patient care.

Payor Mix: Refers to the composition of the types of insurers with which a hospital or physician practice associates. These insurers may include Medicare, Medicaid, and various commercial insurers, such as Blue Cross. Uninsured patients may also comprise part of the payor mix.

Professional Fees: The amount of money paid to a physician for the physician's direct delivery of care to a patient, for the oversight of a procedure, or for the interpretation of a test result.

Quality Improvement Program (QIP): Refers to various methodologies designed to improve the delivery of health-care services. Often focused on process improvement.

Residents: Physicians who have completed medical school and are undergoing a further period of training relative to a specific specialty. Residencies may be for varying periods, from three to seven years or longer, depending on the specialty.

Rules and Regulations: Usually a part of the medical staff bylaws, the rules and regulations are the day-to-day procedures for physicians to admit, care for, and discharge their patients from the hospital. Rules and regulations are usually updated on an annual basis whereas bylaws may be modified less often.

Safe Harbors: Details, under the Stark regulations, the legally acceptable ways in which physicians may refer for various services. Specifically disallows referrals to services where the physician has a financial interest and will benefit from increased utilization of the service.

Sarbanes-Oxley (SOX): This federal act was created to protect investors in public companies by establishing guidelines for corporate oversight, the accuracy of financial disclosures and statements, and the board of director's qualifications and responsibilities. Does not apply to nonprofit organizations, but many have voluntarily agreed to utilize the standards contained in the act.

Stark Regulations: Named for California Congressman Pete Stark, these regulations govern how physicians may self-refer for patient services under the Medicare and Medicaid programs. Designed to prevent referrals to services where the physician will benefit financially, either through ownership or through a contractual relationship.

Technical Fees: The monies paid to a hospital by an insurer for the delivery of a specific procedure or test. See Professional Fees.

Trustee: A legal term to identify a person who has assumed the fiduciary responsibility for the oversight of the operation of a hospital or other nonprofit corporation. The governing body of this type of organization is known as a board of trustees.

Suggestions for Further Reading

I recommend that interested readers continue their education regarding the matters discussed herein. I particularly recommend reading the *Wall Street Journal* on a daily basis, since it is an excellent source of information regarding all facets of medicine and health-care delivery. The paper also offers health-oriented columns and e-mails.

Local business journals are another good source, and most major cities have such a publication. These business journals generally cover the business of health care, both locally and nationally, and may also have available a health-care newsletter via e-mail.

Other journals, such as *Modern Healthcare, Physicians News Digest*, and *Medical Economics*, provide a great deal of useful content and current events and are a regular part of my weekly reading. The Medical Group Management Association offers its members a large amount of reading material that is oriented directly to the operation of a physician practice and can be very helpful when seeking targeted and in-depth information.

www.ingramcontent.com/pod-product-compliance
Lightning Source LLC
Chambersburg PA
CBHW030908180526
45163CB00004B/1752